The Complete Diabetes Diet Book

*Step-by-Step Plan:
How to Reduce Sugar
and Kill Fat*

*Diabetic and Prediabetic
Diet Plan*

ISBN-13: 978-1977766632

ISBN-10: 1977766633

Dedication

I dedicate this book to my sister, Alise, who has been struggling with diabetes all her life, and to all people who want to change their bodies, their health, and their lives.

Introduction

According to a 2016 survey, there is indication that 34.3 million (9.6 percent) people in the United States are affected by diabetes. Diabetes means that the blood glucose or blood sugar in your body is too high. Usually, glucose comes from the food that we eat. An organ called the pancreas makes insulin. Insulin helps glucose get from your blood into your body's cells. Your body's cells carry glucose and turn it into energy required by your body. When you have diabetes, your body has a problem making and using insulin properly. As a result, glucose builds up in your blood and cannot get into your cells. In this case blood glucose will be too high and can be dangerous.

This book will help you to improve your health and increase energy and vitality. Due to a lack of awareness, diabetic people are missing out on a safe way to gain health and energy, and to eliminate toxins from the body in order to maintain a healthy long life.

There are a number of ways to make delicious and nutritious diabetic recipes instead of simply adding a lot of ingredients willy-nilly. So, in order to avoid this, in the following chapters we will discuss each step to control diabetes with easy diet recipes, including health benefits and nutritional information. In addition, you will learn different types of helpful tricks and tips to ensure your diet habits develop as quickly and as easily as possible.

The key to successfully starting a new diet is to do everything within your power to keep a strong mind and dedication to gain health and increase energy by following this diet. Some successful habits to form are to *remind yourself of the wonderful benefits you are going to gain, to follow a routine* and *to reward* yourself with additional food when you have achieved your weekly goal.

Common symptoms of diabetes include:

- Increased urination
- Being thirsty
- Feeling hungry or tired
- Losing weight without any exercise
- Weakness in your body
- Numbness in your feet
- Blurred vision
- Slow healing of wounds and sores

Chapter 1: Causes of Diabetes

Eating lots of sugar is not the only or even the main cause of diabetes. It also depends on your genetic mutations, family heredity, health, ethnicity, damage to your pancreas, various medications, other diseases, hormonal imbalance and environmental factors. For example, as a rule cystic fibrosis creates a thick excretion (mucus) that can cause scarring in the pancreas. This scarring can keep the pancreas from making enough insulin, leading to diabetes.

Another disease, hemochromatosis, causes the body to store excessive iron. If this disease is not treated in time, it leads to damage of the pancreas, among other organs, and causes diabetes. Diabetes can also be inherited through genes passed along in families, which cause the pancreas to produce less insulin.

Some hormone imbalance conditions such as hyperthyroidism, cause the body to produce too much of the thyroid hormone which can lead to insulin resistance and diabetes. Sometimes diabetes is caused by damage to or removal of the pancreas. This reduces or eliminates the number of insulin producing cells, leading to diabetes.

Certain medications or drugs such as anti-seizure drugs, psychiatric drugs, HIV medications, glucocorticoids, niacin, pentamidine, and diuretics can lead to diabetes because these drugs harm beta cells in the pancreas which produce insulin..

Diabetes leads to certain major health problems like stroke, heart attacks, kidney, dental, eye, nerve, and foot problems.

Heart diseases and strokes: Due to diabetes, blood vessels may be damaged which can lead to some heart diseases and also strokes. You can prevent and avoid strokes and heart diseases by properly maintaining your blood pressure, blood glucose and cholesterol levels, and by avoiding smoking.

Hypoglycemia (low blood glucose): Hypoglycemia strikes suddenly when your blood glucose drops too low. This can be prevented by following a proper diet and meal plan, by medications and by balancing physical activities such as walking.

Diabetic neuropathy (nerve damage): Sometimes nerve damage is also caused by diabetes. Most often the nerve damage will be in the feet, limbs and heart. You can feel when your feet become numb for a long time, in which case you must consult your doctor, because, due to decreased blood flow, this can lead to infection and paralysis.

Kidney problems: Kidney problems caused by diabetes are also known as diabetic nephropathy. If diabetes is poorly controlled, it may lead to kidney failure.

Eye problems: Sometimes poorly controlled diabetes will cause nerve damage in the eyes which may lead to temporary blindness, low vision and even permanent blindness. This can be prevented by managing your blood pressure, blood glucose levels, and regular eye checkups.

Urological and sexual problems: The most common disturbance with diabetes is bladder problems like frequent urination, a burning sensation while urinating, and other complications.

Chapter 2: Types of Diabetes

Type 1 diabetes:

In type 1 diabetes your body is unable to make enough insulin. Usually, type 1 diabetes is diagnosed in children and young adults. However, it can show up at any age. People with type 1 diabetes need to take insulin consistently to remain alive.

Causes for type 1 diabetes:

Type 1 diabetes occurs when your immune system and body defenses attack and destroy the beta cells of the pancreas which produce insulin. Research scientists believe that type 1 diabetes is caused mainly by genes and environmental factors such as viral infections. This is called an autoimmune reaction, meaning the body has attacked itself due to following causes:

- Bacterial infection or viral infection
- Chemical toxins formed from food
- A reaction to unidentified components
- Vitamin D deficiency
- Vaccines
- Increased demand for insulin

Symptoms:

- Thirst (above average)
- Tiredness (during day)
- Frequent and uncontrolled urination
- Sudden weight loss
- Genital itchiness

Diagnosis:

If you feel that you may be affected by type 1 diabetes, you should consult your doctor and allow him/her to do blood and urine tests to diagnose diabetes and perhaps suggest some additional tests: ketone test, GAD autoantibodies test, C-peptide test.

Type 2 diabetes:

Type 2 diabetes is one of the most common types of diabetic disorder. If you are suffering from type 2 diabetes it means your body is unable to produce or unable to utilize insulin properly and causes the metabolic disorder of high blood glucose (hyperglycemia). Type 2 diabetes can begin at any age, even in childhood, but mostly occurs in middle-aged and older people.

Type2 diabetes is a serious medical condition that requires anti-diabetic medication and insulin regularly to keep levels of blood sugar under control. Research studies and experiments have shown that type 2 diabetes can be reversed by following a low carbohydrate (low-carb) diet, very-low-calorie diets and basic exercise.

Causes for type 2 diabetes:

Different factors should be considered when evaluating type 2 diabetes. Such as:

- Overweight
- Obesity
- Unhealthy diet
- Physical inactivity

- High cholesterol levels
- Smoking
- Insulin resistance
- Genes and family history

Symptoms:
- Feeling tired after eating a meal
- Feeling hungry again after a short time (polyphagia)
- Frequent urination, especially at night (polyuria)
- Abnormal thirst (polydipsia)
- Blurred vision
- Itchy skin, especially around the genitals
- Taking a long time to heal (cuts and wounds)
- Yeast infections
- Skin disorders (like psoriasis and acanthosis nigricans)
- Sudden loss of muscle mass (weight loss)
- Nausea
- Fatigue
- Dizziness

Treatment: Using regular diabetes medications, healthy diet, physical activity and exercise, controlled blood pressure levels and cholesterol levels.

Gestational diabetes:

Gestational diabetes develops in some women while they are pregnant. Most of the time, this kind of diabetes goes away after the baby is born. However, if you've had gestational diabetes, you have a greater chance of getting type 2 diabetes later in life. Sometimes the diabetes that occurs during pregnancy is really type 2 diabetes. Gestational diabetes may predispose to other health issues in both moms and infants.

Causes for gestational diabetes:

Gestational diabetes happens when the body is unable to make the extra insulin needed during pregnancy. Insulin, a hormone made by the pancreas, facilitates the body's use of glucose for energy and helps manage the blood glucose levels.

During pregnancy, the body makes special hormones and goes through other modifications, e.g., weight gain. Because of these modifications, the body's cells don't use insulin properly — a circumstance known as insulin resistance. All pregnant women have a little insulin resistance throughout pregnancy, but most can produce enough insulin to overcome the insulin resistance, however a few cannot. These women develop gestational diabetes.

Being obese or overweight is associated with gestational diabetes. Women who are obese or overwight may in fact already have insulin resistance when they get pregnant. Gaining too much weight in the course of pregnancy can also be an effect. Having a family history of diabetes makes it more likely that a woman will experience gestational diabetes, indicating that genes play a major role.

Symptoms:

Gestational diabetes regularly has no symptoms, or they can be mild — being thirstier than usual or more frequent urination. Gestational diabetes is occasionally associated with the hormonal changes of pregnancy that make the body much less able to use insulin. Genes and extra weight may additionally play a role as mentioned.

Diagnosis:

Testing for gestational diabetes generally takes place between 24 and 28 weeks of pregnancy. If you have an increased risk of developing gestational diabetes, your doctor may test for diabetes at some time during the first few visits after you become pregnant.

Tests include the glucose challenge test and the oral glucose tolerance test (OGTT). If the results of the glucose challenge test look suspicious , you'll return for an OGTT to confirm the diagnosis of gestational diabetes.

Prediabetes:

Prediabetes is a situation in which blood glucose or A1C levels are slight elevated above normal, but not sufficiently elevated for a diagnosis of diabetes. Nowa-days in the United States, prediabetes is becoming more common. According to a U.S. Department of Health and Human Services survey, a minimum of 84.1 million U.S. adults have prediabetes. People with prediabetes have a higher risk of developing type 2 diabetes and cardiovascular diseases (CVD), which create health problems like heart attacks and/or strokes.

Causes of prediabetes:

Insulin resistance increases the risk of developing prediabetes. Prediabetes usually occurs in people who already have insulin resistance. The main problem in prediabetes is that the beta cells can't produce enough insulin to overcome insulin resistance and, thus, glucose levels increase above the normal level. Once a person gets prediabetes, if the beta cells continue to decline, it mayl finally lead to type 2 diabetes, with the results seen from hyperglycemia (high blood glucose): damaged nerves, blindness, blood vessel damage, heart disease, stroke, lower-limb amputations and kidney failure.

Symptoms:

Prediabetes typically has no signs. Even without signs and symptoms, health care and fitness professionals can often notice prediabetic people by their physical characteristics. Prediabetics may have dark patches of skin and noticeable pores, usually at the back of the neck, or darkish rings around their necks, and dark patches may also appear on the knees, elbows, armpits and knuckles. This is known as *acanthosis nigricans*.

Diagnosis:

Health care centers use blood tests to determine whether a person has prediabetes. Health care labs analyze blood to ensure best results and nowadays new portable devices are available to measure glucose: for example, finger-stick devices used to find high blood glucose levels. Prediabetes may be detected with one of the following blood tests:

- A1C test
- Fasting plasma glucose (FPG) test
- Oral glucose tolerance test (OGTT)

Chapter 3: List of Foods Good for Diabetics

Firstly, there is no need to worry that having diabetes makes you miss out on nice tasty food. In fact, you can have your favorite food items but in small portions. Nutritional food and physical activities are essential parts of a healthy lifestyle when you have diabetes. To become extra energetic and active, the need to make adjustments in what you consume and drink might be tough in the beginning but later you will feel better.

To help you, our team created a diabetes meal plan (see below) that meets your needs and likes. You just need to follow the step by step procedure to make delicious and yummy meals.

VEGETABLES	Celery, Tomatoes, Bell Peppers, Onions, Leeks, Kohlrabi, Green Onions, Eggplants, Cauliflower, Broccoli, Asparagus, Cucumber, Cabbage, Brussels Sprouts, Artichokes, Okra, Avocados
GREEN LEAFY VEGETABLES	Lettuce, Spinach, Collard Greens, Kale, Beet Top, Mustard Greens, Dandelion, Swiss Chard, Watercress, Turnip Greens, Seaweeds, Endive, Arugula (Rocket), Bok Choy, Rapini, Chicory, Radicchio
ROOT VEGETABLES	Carrots, Beets, Turnips, Parsnips, Rutabaga, Sweet Potatoes, Radish, Jerusalem Artichokes, Yams, Cassava
WINTER SQUASH	Butternut Squash, Spaghetti Squash Acorn Squash, Pumpkin, Buttercup Squash.
SUMMER SQUASH	Zucchini, Yellow Summer Squash, Yellow Crookneck Squash
FRUIT	Apples, Pomegranates, Pears, Avocado, Guava, Berries (Strawberry, Cranberry, Blueberry, Blackberry, Raspberry), Plantains, Grapefruit, Peaches, Nectarines, Plums, Pineapple, Papaya, Cantaloupe, Cherries, Apricot, Honeydew Melon, Kiwi, Lemon, Lime, Lychee, Tangerine, Coconut, Figs, Olives, Passion Fruit, Persimmon

NUTS & SEEDS	Pistachios, Brazil Nuts, Sunflower Seeds, Sesame Seeds, Chia Seeds, Flax Seeds, Pumpkin Seeds (Pepitas), Pecans, Walnuts, Pine Nuts, Macadamia Nuts, Chestnuts, Cashews, Almonds, Hazelnuts
HERBS	Parsley, Thyme, Lavender, Mint, Basil, Rosemary, Chives, Tarragon, Oregano, Sage, Dill, Bay Leaves, Coriander
SPICES & OTHERS	Ginger, Garlic, Onions, Black Pepper, Hot Peppers, Star Anise, Fennel Seeds, Mustard Seeds, Cayenne Pepper, Cumin, Turmeric, Cinnamon, Nutmeg, Paprika, Vanilla, Cloves, Chilies, Horseradish, Oatmeal, Eggs, Soy, Yogurt

Chapter 4: List of Foods to Avoid

Why is sugar bad?

The vast majority of us think of "sugar" as what we sweeten coffee or espresso with, but in chemical terms, sugar is only the building blocks of carbohydrates in our bodies. Research studies confirm that the connection between sugar and weight gain is tremendous. Sugar is the one of the main causes of every modern health problem.

- Sugar must be converted by the liver before it can be utilized for energy by your body's cells It has a similar effect on the liver as alcohol.
- Sugar increases uric acid production in the body, which is one cause of kidney stones.
- The abundance of sugar alone can cause every one of the issues related with the metabolic disorders (heart disease, obesity, diabetes).

DAIRY	**Milk, Butter, Buttermilk, Kefir, Cream, Ghee, Ice Cream, Powdered Milk, Cottage Cheese, The milk of all Mammals**
SUGAR	Avoid Sugar (Try Artificial Sweeteners)
PROCESSED FOOD	Frozen Meals, Fast Food, Sweets
OTHERS	French fries, potato chips, Sodas, Bacon, Processed grains, White bread, Fried items, Pickles

Chapter 5: Tips and Tricks to Keep Diabetes under Control

You can manage your diabetes and maintain a healthier life each day by following some simple steps, such as managing your blood glucose levels, also known as blood sugar. Managing your blood glucose, blood pressure and cholesterol also prevents health issues that arise while having diabetes. Below are mentioned some self-care steps to help manage your diabetes

- Manage your A1C test.
- Manage your blood pressure.
- Manage your cholesterol.
- Stop smoking.
- Make a diabetes meal plan.
- Increase physical activity.
- Take your medicine ontime.
- Check your blood glucose levels.

Manage your A1C test: The A1C test tells your average blood glucose level in your body during the last three months. The main intention of the A1C test is to help people with diabetes keep their A1C below 7 percent.

Manage your blood pressure: The blood pressure measurement should be less than 140/90 mm Hg. Controlling your diabetes will help lower this reading.

Manage your cholesterol: There are two types of cholesterol in your blood, the LDL and the HDL. LDL is bad cholesterol; at high levels it will clog your blood vessels and lead to heart attacks or strokes. The HDL, on the other hand, is good cholesterol; it will help remove bad cholesterol from your blood vessels.

Stop smoking: Avoiding smoking is especially important for people with diabetes because both smoking and diabetes narrow blood vessels.making your heart work harder and increasing your blood pressure. So, cigarettes aren't a safe choice for diabetic people. Some of the advantages of avoiding smoking are:

- Less risk of heart attacks, stroke, nerve diseases, kidney problems, diabetic eye disease and amputation
- Improvement in cholesterol and blood pressure levels in the body
- Improvement in blood circulation in the body
- Improvement in physical activity.

Perfect a diabetes meal plan: Try to make a proper diabetes meal plan with the help of your health center dietician. Following a proper meal plan will assist in controlling your blood glucose, blood pressure and cholesterol. Try to choose foods which will be lower in calories, saturated fat, trans fats, sugar, and salt. If you are overweight or obese, ask your health center team to create and make a proper weight-loss plan to keep diabetes under control.

Physical activity: Make up your mind to do regular physical activity at least 30 minutes per day. Brisk walks and swimming are the best options for diabetics. If you are busy, just ask your health center for simple home exercises to keep you physically energetic and active throughout the day.

Take your medicine on time: Don't forget to take your medicine on time to avoid instant health problems in fluctuations of your blood glucose and blood pressure. Also, contact your doctor immediately if you have any side effects such as numbness and blurred vision.

Basic exercises

With any diet, training is the key to establishing a new habit, For example, 10-15 minutes of physical exercise per day will help a lot. Let's look at some of the important changes you should make to contribute to losing weight faster when you are on a diet.

Park and walk: I think you have already heard about this technique, and I am 100% sure that this works. Instead of parking in front of your office or workplace, park a little further away . . . in the next parking lot, say, Clearly this makes you walk and helps improve blood flow in your body.

Mostly prefer the stairs: Instead of using the elevator in your office or any other place, use the stairs which contracts your muscles and keeps your joints, ligaments, and bones limber . . . and it will burn more calories.

Take advantage of shopping: If you don't have a big shopping list, then this is the right time to spurn the shopping cart. Keep shopping bags that you can carry handy. Carrying the heavy grocery items with your hands is a great workout and at the same time you will be finishing your shopping.

Stretch yourself: Sitting in front of your desk or computer for hours is extremely sluggish for the body, but there are lots of ways that you can work out while sitting. One the best ways is to flex and contract your legs at regular intervals, and whenever you go to the toilet or for coffee, stretch your whole body. Upgrade to using a stability ball instead of sitting in a regular chair.

Chapter 6: Glycemic Indexes and Food Chart

What is the glycemic index (GI)

The Glycemic Index (GI) is a measurement performed on carbohydrate-containing foods and their effect on our blood sugar. GI is a new way of effectively analyzing foods. Previously, meal plans designed to improve blood sugar analyzed the whole quantity of carbohydrates (which include sugars and starches) included in the meals themselves. GI is going beyond this approach, looking at the effect of meals on our real blood sugar. In other words, as opposed to counting the total amount of carbohydrates in unconsumed foods, GI measures the actual impact of those eaten ingredients on our blood sugar levels. In the table below, we classified all food items as low, medium, or high in their GI values.

Health benefits

For 15 years now, low-GI diets have been connected to a decreased threat of Type 2 diabetes, cardiovascular disease, metabolic syndromes, stroke, kidney diseases, gallstones, kindney tubes defects, formation of uterine fibroids, breast cancers and pancreas. Taking advantage of those health benefits may be as easy as sticking with whole, natural foods which can be either low or very low in their GI value. Checkout the table below for selected GI food items listed by their GI value.

High GI (>70)		Medium GI (56-69)		Low GI (0-55)	
FRUITS					
Watermelon	72	Pineapple	66	Apples	38
		Apricots	57	Bananas	54
		Cantaloupe	65	Blueberries	50
		Figs	63	Cranberries	52
		Papaya	60	Grapefruit	25
		Mangoes	56	Grapes	46
		Raisins	64	Kiwifruit	53
		Fruit cocktail	56	Lemons/Limes	28
				Oranges	44
				Pears	38
				Plums & Prunes	39
				Raspberries	32
				Strawberries	40

VEGETABLES

Potatoes	83	Beets	64		
Parsnips	97	Corn	60	Carrots	39
		Sweet Potatoes	56		
				Beet Greens	15
				Eggplant	15
				Garlic	16
				Leeks	15
				Bell Peppers	40
				Green Peas	22
				Bok Choy	54
				Onions	10
				Broccoli	15
				Sea Vegetables	49
				Brussels Sprouts	52
				Winter Squash	54
				Cabbage	48
				Cauliflower	20
				Celery	
				Collard Greens	
				Cucumbers	15
				Fennel (Bulb)	32
				Green Beans	15
				Kale	15

				Mustard Greens	18
				Olives	22
				Yam	51
				All Lettuce	15
				Spinach	15
				Summer Squash	52
				Swiss Chard	20
				Tomatoes	15
				Turnip Greens	16
Beans & Legumes					
Broad Beans	79			Soybeans	16
				Black Beans	41
				Tofu	22
				Dried Peas	22
				Tempeh	25
				Garbanzo Beans	44
				Kidney Beans	52
				Lentils	52
				Lima Beans	52
				Navy Beans	48
				Pinto Beans	52
Nuts & Seeds & Sweets					
Dates	103	Popcorn	55	Almonds	30
Jelly Beans	80	Mars Bar	64	Flaxseeds	32

Corn Chips	74	Chocolate	49	Sesame Seeds	35
		Sucrose	65	Peanuts	15
				Pumpkin Seeds	25
				Sunflower Seeds	35
				Walnuts	15

Seafood & Meats

				Scallops	43
				Cod	18
				Salmon	18
				Sardines	18
				Shrimp	18
				Tuna	18
				Beef	20
				Chicken	20
				Lamb	20
				Turkey	20

Dairy

		Ice-Cream	61	Cheese	34
				Eggs	24
				Cow Milk	27
				Yogurt	14

Cereal Grains

Millet	71	Brown Rice	56	Pearl Barley	25
		Wild Rice	57	Rye	34
		White Rice	58	Wheat Kernels	41
		Barley	66	Rice (Instant)	46

Herbs & Spices

		(Parboiled)	
		Chili Pepper	10
		Cilantro & Coriander Seeds	10
		Cinnamon	12
		Cloves	10
		Cumin Seeds	12
		Dill	10
		Ginger	15
		Mustard Seeds	10
		Oregano	10
		Parsley	10
		Peppermint	12
		Rosemary	12
		Sage	10
		Thyme	10
		Turmeric	10

Breakfast Cereals

Golden Grahams	71	Oat Bran	55	All-Bran	42
Puffed Wheat	74	Muesli	56	Porridge	49
Weetabix	77	Mini Wheats (Whole meal)	57		
Rice Krispies	82	Shredded Wheat	69		
Cornflakes	83				

Breads

White Bread	71	Pita Bread, White	57	Multi Grain Bread	48
White Rolls	73	Pizza, Cheese	60	Whole Grain	50
Baguette	95	Hamburger Bun	61		
		Rye-Flour Bread	63		
		Whole Meal Bread	69		

Beverages

				Soy Milk	30
				Apple Juice	41
				Carrot Juice	45
				Pineapple Juice	46
				Grapefruit Juice	48
				Orange Juice	52

Bakery Items

Waffles	76	Danish Pastry	59	
Doughnut	76	Muffin(Un-sweetened)	62	
		Cake, Tart & Angel Food	65	
		Croissant	67	

Pasta

Brown Rice Pasta	92	Spaghetti (Durum Wheat)	56	Fettuccine	32
		Macaroni Cheese	64	Vermicelli	35
				Spaghetti (Whole Wheat)	37
				Ravioli	39
				Macaroni	45

Soups

		Black Bean Soup	64	Tomato Soup	38
		Green Pea Soup	66	Lentil Soup	44

Chapter 7: Delicious Diabetes Recipes

Breakfast Recipes

Recipe 1: Avocado Omelet

- Preparation Time: 25 minutes
- Total servings: 3

Ingredients

- Large eggs 5
- Tomato 1
- Avocado 1
- Olive oil 1 tbsp.
- Green pepper 2
- Spring onions 1 oz.
- Watercress, chopped, 2 tbsp.
- Salt and pepper to taste

Preparation Method

- Dice all vegetables which are listed above (except avocado).
- Fry vegetables in a pan with olive oil .
- Once rinds are crispy, mix together well. Seasoned as needed.
- Once spring onions are translucent, add chopped watercress to the pan and mix everything together and allow it to cook for 2 minutes.
- Add eggs and mix everything together and let it cook like an omelet.
- Before serving, just add avocado cubes and mix. Enjoy the delicious taste.

Recipe 2: Morning Almond Bars

- Preparation Time: 15 minutes
- Total servings: 20

Ingredients

- Almond butter 1 cup
- Pumpkin purée 1 cup
- Ground cinnamon 1 tbsp.
- Peanuts, chopped, 1 oz.
- Pumpkin spices
- Protein powder 2 oz.
- Coconut butter 2 oz.
- Ghee 2 tbsp.

Preparation Method

1. Hold aside 8x8 inch square baking tray with aluminum foil. In a large bowl, add melted coconut butter, pumpkin spices protein powder and mix well.
2. Add ghee and combine well without lumps. Pour the mixture into the already prepared pan and spread evenly then sprinkle chopped peanuts.
3. Cover with wax paper and using your hands spread the batter evenly into the pan. Remove wax paper and place the mixture in the refrigerator for 3 hours.
4. Use a sharp knife to cut into 25 equal squares and enjoy the delicious taste.

Recipe 3: Pumpkin Bread

- Preparation Time: 80 minutes
- Total servings: 12

Ingredients

Bread:

- Almond flour 7 oz.
- Pumpkin spice 2 tsp.
- Cream of tartar 1 tsp.
- Baking soda ¼ tsp.
- Lemon zest 1 tbsp.
- Juice of half a lemon
- Ghee 2 oz.
- Large eggs 4
- Erythritol 3 oz.
- Cinnamon 1 tsp.
- Pumpkin purée 5 oz.

Topping:

- Small egg 1
- Erythritol 1½ oz.
- Cinnamon ½ tsp.
- Pumpkins purée 3½ oz.
- Lemon zest 1 tbsp.
- Pinch of salt

Preparation Method

1. Preheat the oven to 300°F. In a large bowl, add almond flour, cinnamon, pumpkin spice, cream of tartar, baking soda and mix well. Add eggs, ghee, erythritol, and cinnamon and combine well.

2. Add a spoon of pumpkin purée and mix well (fresh pumpkin purée gives a better taste than canned purée).
3. Now, add juice of half a lemon and the zest, and mix. In another bowl, prepare the topping by mixing together all topping ingredients.
4. Spoon the bread batter into a suitable baking dish and distribute evenly using a ladle. Add a layer using half of the topping mixture on top of the bread batter and spread evenly.
5. Mix the remaining half of the topping mixture with the pumpkin purée. Gently spoon the pumpkin mixture on top and spread evenly. Transfer to the preheated oven and bake for 60 minutes. Make sure that bread does not burn on top.
6. Carefully remove from the baking dish, slice into 12 pieces and enjoy.

Recipe 4: Lemon Bread

- Preparation Time: 15 minutes
- Total servings: 2

Ingredients

Bread

- Stevia 2 tbsp.
- Ghee 2 tbsp.
- Egg 1
- Egg yolks 2
- Lemon juice 2 tsp.
- Vanilla extracts 1 tsp.
- Almond flour ½ oz.
- Baking powder ½ tsp.
- Flax flour 2 tsp.
- Pinch of salt

Blackberry Glaze

- Butter 2 tbsp.
- Blackberries 1 oz.
- Erythritol 3 tbsp.

Preparation Method

1. Preheat the oven to 350°F. In a mixing bowl, add all bread ingredients together and mix well until it forms a nice batter.
2. Line a baking sheet with parchment paper and place the batter on it (if desired, you can create your own bread loaf shape).
3. Place in the preheated oven and bake for 10 minutes. Let it cool for 5 minutes.
4. Meanwhile, prepare the glaze by adding all ingredients in a small bowl and mix using a hand mixer.
5. Put this glaze in the refrigerator for a minimum of 30 minutes. Using a spoon, gently glaze your bread and enjoy.

Recipe 5: Creamy Oatmeal

- Preparation Time: 15 minutes
- Total servings: 6

Ingredients

- Crushed Pecans $7/8$ cup
- Flax seeds 2 oz.
- Chia seeds 2 oz.
- Riced cauliflower 2 oz.
- Almond milk 2 cups
- Protein powder 1 tbsp.
- Cinnamon 1 tsp
- Maple flavoring 1 tsp
- Vanilla extract ½ tsp
- Nutmeg ¼ tsp
- Allspice ¼ tsp
- Powdered erythritol 1 oz.
- Liquid stevia 10 drops

Preparation Method

1. Mix flax and chia seeds in a small cup and keep aside. In a food processor, add riced cauliflower and protein powder, and keep aside
2. Toast the raw pecans in a pan (before you toast, smash pecans into small pieces)
3. In another pan, add coconut milk and boil until it is cooked well
4. Decrease heat under the pan and add cinnamon, maple flavoring, vanilla, nutmeg and allspice to the coconut milk. Add powdered erythritol and stevia, stir well
5. Next add flax seeds and chia seeds to the milk mixture and mix well. Heat, stirring often,until it starts to thicken
6. Add pecans, and mix together well and to make it a bit thicker and enjoy the taste

Lunch Recipes

Recipe 6: Chicken Bone Soup

- Preparation Time: 3 hours 10 minutes
- Serving per Recipe: 5

Ingredients

- Chicken bones 1 lb.
- Onion Powder 1 tsp.
- Garlic Powder 1 tsp.
- Ginger powder 1 tsp.
- Chili powder ½ tsp.
- Ghee 2 oz.
- Squash 1 oz.
- Soy sauce 2 oz.
- Chicken broth 3 cups
- Cream cheese 2 oz.
- Cumin powder 1 tsp.
- Salt and Pepper to taste

Preparation Method

1. Break the chicken bones into chunks and drop them in a pot and add all the rest of the ingredients to the cooking pot except the cream cheese.
2. Set cooking pot on heat for 60 minutes and cook completely. Once everything is cooked, remove the chicken from the cooking pot and shred using a fork.
3. Add cream cheese to the cooking pot. Using an immersion blender, emulsify all of the liquids together (removethe bones before you do this). This will keep the soup from separating while you are eating
4. Place the chicken back into the cooking pot. Taste and season with extra salt, pepper, cumin and soy sauce, if needed. Serve and enjoy the taste.

Recipe 7: Baked Eggs with Kale

- Preparation Time: 25 minutes
- Total servings: 4

Ingredients

- Olive oil 2 tsp.
- Diced shallots 1 oz.
- Kale 3 cups
- Large eggs 4
- Salt and ground pepper to taste
- Blue cheese 1 oz.
- Mascarpone 1 oz.
- Garlic cloves 3, minced
- Grated coconut 1 oz.

Preparation Method

1. Preheat oven to 400°F. Grease 4 ramekins with butter. Heat a large pan over medium heat. Add ghee and shallots and cook 2 minutes.
2. Add kale, salt, pepper, water and boil until the kale wilts— about 3 minutes. Mix in blue cheese, mascarpone and remove from the heat.
3. Divide the wilted kale evenly into the 4 ramekins and make a depression in the middle of each. Drop an egg into the depression in each dish and season with grated coconut, minced garlic, salt and pepper.
4. Place the ramekins on a baking sheet and bake until the whites are set and the yolks are firm around the edges, but still soft in the middle— about 15 minutes. Serve immediately.

Recipe 8: Mushroom Meal

- Preparation Time: 15 minutes
- Total servings: 1

Ingredients

- Egg 1
- Mushrooms 6 oz.
- Sweet potato, cubed, 2 oz.
- Red bell pepper 1 oz.
- Ghee 1 tbsp.
- Salt and pepper to taste
- Fresh sage 1 tbsp.

Preparation Method

1. In a small pan, sauté the mushrooms with ghee and season with salt, pepper. Keep aside.
2. Roast the bacon, sweet potato cubes, and red pepper and keep aside. In the same pan, make an omelet with the egg and garnish with freshly chopped sage.
3. Finally, place all items on a serving plate and enjoy.

Recipe 9: Salmon with Mint Paste

- Preparation Time: 15 minutes
- Total Servings: 2

Ingredients

- Salmon fillets 1 lb.
- Mint paste 3 tbsp. (see step #1 below)
- Mustard ½ tsp.
- Thyme ¼ tsp.
- Ghee 1 tbsp.
- Salt and pepper to taste

Preparation Method

1. Preheat the oven to 350°F. Place macadamia nuts, mint, maple syrup, your spices and mustard in food processor and make a paste.
2. Heat a pan and add ghee. Sear the salmon fillets on each side for about 3 minutes. Add the mint paste to the top of each salmon fillet.
3. Once they are seared, transfer them to the oven and bake for about 10 minutes. Serve with some fresh baby kale and smoked paprika to add extra flavor.

Recipe 10: Creamy Vegetable Soup

- Preparation Time: 5 minutes
- Total Servings: 1

Ingredients

- Vegetable broth 1½ cup
- Mixed vegetables 1 oz.
- Bouillon cubes 2
- Olive oil 1 tbsp.
- Large eggs 2 (hard boiled)
- Rosemary 2 tbsp.
- Mascarpone cheese 1 oz.
- Chili paste ½ tsp.
- Garlic paste ½ tsp.

Preparation Method

1. Place a pan over medium heat and add vegetable broth, vegetables, bouillon cubes, and olive oil.
2. Bring the broth to a boil and stir everything together, then add the chili paste and garlic paste, and stir again. Turn the stove off.
3. Chop the boiled eggs and add them to the steaming broth. Add mascarpone cheese and stir together well. Let the soup sit for a moment and add chopped rosemary leaves. Serve up some awesome tasting soup in just 5 minutes!

Dinner Recipes

Recipe 11: Chicken Pumpkin Zoodles

- Preparation Time: 20 minutes
- Total servings: 2

Ingredients

- Chicken breast 3½ oz.
- Olive oil 1 tbsp.
- Ghee 1 tbsp.
- Curry powder ½ tsp.
- Spring onion 1 stalk
- Garlic 1 clove
- Large egg 1
- Sprouts 1 oz.
- Pumpkin 3½ oz.
- Soy sauce 1 tsp.
- Fish sauce ½ tsp.
- Pepper ¼ tsp.
- Lime juice 1 tsp.
- Green chili pepper 1
- Cilantro 1 tbsp.
- Salt and pepper to taste

Preparation Method

1. Season the chicken with curry powder, salt and pepper and set aside.
2. Prepare the sauce by combining the soy sauce and fish sauce.
3. Finely chop the spring onion and garlic. Make zoodles out of pumpkin (use a spiralizer)
4. Fry the seasoned chicken with olive oil until brown.
5. In a pan, melt ghee and sauté the chopped spring onion until fragrant. Add the garlic and egg to the pan.
6. Add sprouts and zoodles and mix everything well

together and continue cooking until the sprouts and zoodles are tender.

7. Cut the fried chciken into pieces. Add the chicken to the pan and squeeze some lemon juice on top. Enjoy.

Recipe 12: Pepperoni and Cauliflower "Rice"

- Preparation Time: 20 minutes
- Total servings: 4

Ingredients

- Riced cauliflower 1 lb.
- Pepperoni 8½ oz.
- Jalapeño peppers 3 oz.
- Dried red chili 1
- Fresh turnip greens 1 tbsp.
- Fresh rosemary 1 tbsp.
- Olive oil 2 tbsp.
- Ghee 2 tbsp
- Salt and pepper to taste

Preparation Method

1. Grate cauliflower and make "rice" from it. Set aside.
2. Slice pepperoni, jalapeño peppers, and dried red chili and keep aside.
3. Place a large skillet over medium heat and add ghee. When ghee is hot, add peppers, chili, turnip greens and pepperoni. Cook until slightly browned.
4. Add the cauliflower "rice" and cook for 10 minutes, season with salt, pepper. Add finely chopped rosemary and enjoy the flavors.

Recipe 13: Salmon Wraps

- Preparation Time: 15 minutes
- Total servings: 2

Ingredients

- Large eggs 3
- Avocado 3½ oz.
- Smoked salmon 2 oz.
- Fresh dill 2 tbsp.
- Spring onion 2 tbsp.
- Mascarpone cheese 2 oz
- Ghee 1 tbsp.
- Salt and pepper to taste

Preparation Method

1. Whisk eggs, salt and pepper in a small bowl, add mascarpone cheese with chopped dill and keep aside.
2. Place a pan over medium heat and add ghee. When ghee is hot, add egg mixture and cook for 1 minute, flip over and cook for one minute longer.
3. Meanwhile, slice the smoked salmon and avocado and set aside. Slide the unfolded omelet onto a plate, add sliced salmon and avocado, and fold into a wrap.

Recipe 14: Dandelion Omelet

- Preparation Time: 40 minutes
- Total servings: 4

Ingredients

- Ghee 1 tbsp.
- Onion 1 oz.
- Dandelion greens 10 oz.
- Large eggs 8
- Sea salt 1 tsp.
- Goat cheese 2 oz
- Mascarpone 1 oz
- Black pepper ½ tsp.

Preparation Method

1. Preheat the oven to 350°F and place a pan over medium heat. Add ghee and when it is hot, add onion and cook until it becomes soft.
2. Add dandelion greens and cook for 2 minutes. Place aside. In a bowl, mix eggs, goat cheese, mascarpone, salt, pepper and add to dandelion mixture.
3. Using a blender, blend the mixture and pour into a pan. Put the pan in the preheated oven for 30 minutes and enjoy.

Recipe 15: Summer Vegetable Stew

- Preparation Time: 40 minutes
- Total Servings: 5

Ingredients

- Vegetable mix 1 lb.
- Ghee 2 tbsp.
- Garlic powder 1 tsp.
- Ginger powder 1 tsp.
- Tomato purée 1½ oz.
- All spice 1½ tbsp.
- Paprika 1½ tsp.
- Salt and pepper to taste
- Diced tomatoes 7 oz.
- Coconut milk 1 cup
- Cashew paste 1 tbsp.
- Mascarpone
- Parsley 1½ tbsp.

Preparation Method

1. Cut vegetable mix into bite-sized pieces and season with salt, pepper, garlic, and ginger and mix well.
2. Add canned diced tomatoes and tomato paste, mix well again. Next add coconut milk and cashew paste and mix well.
3. Cook for 25 minutes on medium heat., Add coconut cream, mix thoroughly and cook for 10 minutes more. Before serving, add ghee, grated mascarpone and enjoy the taste.

Salad Recipes

Recipe 16: Green Herb Salad

- Preparation Time: 10 minutes
- Total servings: 2

Ingredients

- Mixed greens 1 oz. (spinach, kale, collards)
- Fresh herbs 1 oz. (Mint, Thyme)
- Roasted pine nuts 1 oz.
- Vinaigrette 1½ tbsp.
- Parmesan cheese 1 tbsp.
- Ghee 1 tbsp.
- Bacon 1 oz
- Salt and pepper to taste

Preparation Method

1. Cook bacon until crisp. Place the greens and herbs in a container that can be shaken.
2. Crumble bacon over the greens, and add the salt, pepper and vinaigrette. Shake the container with a lid.
3. Add the pine nuts, Parmesan and ghee, and shake once again to coat everything well. Serve and enjoy the taste.

Recipe 17: Veggie Salad

- Preparation Time: 12 minutes
- Total Servings: 2

Ingredients

- Fresh tomato 1
- Vegetable mix 2 oz. (Cucumber, Carrot, Bell pepper, Beet)
- Fresh mozzarella cheese 6 oz.
- Turnip greens 1 tbsp.
- Fresh basil 1½ tbsp.
- Olive oil 3 tbsp.
- Vinegar 1 tbsp.
- Mascarpone 1 oz.
- Fresh black pepper to taste
- Himalaya salt to taste

Preparation Method

1. In a food processor, put chopped fresh basil, turnip leaves and olive oil and process to make a paste.
2. Slice tomato into 1/4″ slices. You should be able to get at least 6 slices from the tomato.
3. Cut Mozzarella and mascarpone into slices. Assemble salad by layering tomato, mozzarella, mascarpone,and the paste.
4. Season with salt, pepper, and olive oil and enjoy the taste.

Recipe 18: Macadamia Green Salad

- Preparation Time: 10 minutes
- Total servings: 1

Ingredients

- Mixed greens 2 oz.
- Roasted macadamia nuts 1 oz.
- Vinaigrette 4 tsp.
- Parsley 1 tbsp.
- Bacon 2 oz.
- Salt and pepper (as desired)

Preparation Method

1. Cook bacon until crisp. Put the greens in a container that can be shaken.
2. Crumble bacon over the greens , add the vinaigrette, and shake the container with a lid.
3. Add the salt and pepper, the nuts and the chopped parsley and shake once again to coat with dressing. Serve and enjoy.

Recipe 19: Avocado Salad

- Preparation Time: 10 minutes
- Total servings: 6

Ingredients

- Large hard boiled eggs 4
- Avocado 5-6 oz.
- Greek yogurt 1 tbsp.
- Salt ½ tsp.
- Ghee 1 tbsp.
- Nuts 1 oz.
- Mayonnaise 1 oz.
- Mascarpone 2 oz.
- Ground pepper to taste

Preparation Method

- Combine avocado, mayonnaise, yogurt, salt and pepper. Combine with mashed eggs and adjust salt and pepper as needed.
- Sprinkle with chopped nuts, ghee, and mascarpone cheese and enjoy the taste.

Recipe 20: Ham Salad

- Preparation Time: 65 minutes
- Total servings: 3

Ingredients

- Tuna 1 lb.
- Soy sauce 1 tbsp.
- Ghee 1 tbsp.
- Water 1 tbsp.
- Garlic paste 1 tsp.
- Vinegar 2 tsp.
- Lemon juice 1 tbsp.
- Chopped cilantro 1 tbsp.

Preparation Method

1. Cut the tuna and set aside. For the marinade. combine soy sauce, ghee, water, garlic paste and vinegar.
2. Mix the ham and marinade mixture in a bowl and keep aside for 30 minutes. Preheat oven to 350°F Place the ham on a baking tray covered with parchment paper and bake for 30 minutes.
3. Once ham is ready, sprinkle with the cilantro, and lemon juice. Enjoy.

Snack Recipes

Recipe 21: Broccoli Biscuits

- Preparation Time: 30 minutes
- Total servings: 12

Ingredients

- Almond flour 1½ cup
- Broccoli florets 1½ lb.
- Olive oil 2 oz.
- Large eggs 2
- Salt to taste
- Ginger powder 1 tsp.
- Baking soda ½ tsp.
- Apple cider ½ tsp.
- Cheddar cheese 2 oz.
- Mascarpone 1 oz.
- Peppers

Preparation Method

1. Preheat the oven to 375°F. Finely chop the broccoli florets.
2. In a large bowl, mix well the almond flour, salt, peppers, ginger powder, baking soda. Add eggs and olive oil ghee. Mix until a dough forms.
3. Add the broccoli to the mixture. Combine everything with your hands. Grate cheddar and mascarpone into the dough. Mix everything with your hands until the cheese is evenly distributed.
4. Place a nonstick silpat on a cookie sheet, so the biscuits will not stick as they bake. Form biscuits

from the dough. Bake for 15 minutes or until they begin to flatten.

5. Turn them over and continue baking for about 5 minutes longer, and then turn the oven heat to broil and brown the biscuits for 3 minutes. Let them cool for 2 minutes before you enjoy them.

Recipe 22: Wild Mushroom Bowl

- Preparation Time: 35 minutes
- Total servings: 4

Ingredients

- Macadamia nuts ½ cup
- Parsley 2 cups
- Garlic paste 2 tsp.
- Lemon juice 2 tbsp.
- Salt and pepper to taste
- Wild mushrooms 1 lb.
- Cauliflower florets 2 oz.
- Ghee 1 tbsp.
- Mascarpone 1 oz.
- Kale 1 bunch

Preparation Method

1. Soak the macadamia nuts overnight in water. Drain and add the macadamia nuts, parsley, garlic paste, lemon juice, salt, and pepper to a food processor and process until smooth.
2. Cook the cauliflower in a small pan over medium heat for 10 minutes and set aside. Place a large skillet over medium heat with the ghee and add

mushrooms, season with salt and pepper and cook for 10 minutes stirring occasionally until all the water has evaporated and the mushrooms begin to brown Tranfer to a bowl and set aside.

3. Add kale to the same pan and cook for 2 minutes or until kale is wilted and a bright green color.
4. Finally, combine the cauliflower, the wild mushrooms, mascarpone, and kale, and divide between 4 bowls. Top each bowl with a tablespoon of the macadamia nut "pesto" and enjoy the delicious taste.

Recipe 23: Harvested Avocado Bowl

- Preparation Time: 20 minutes
- Total servings: 2

Ingredients

- Arugula 1 cup
- Brussels Sprouts 1 cup (sautéed)
- Avocado ½ (sliced)
- Ghee 1 tbsp.
- Tahini sauce 1 tbsp.
- Salt and Pepper to taste

Preparation Method

1. Sauté sprouts in ghee for approximately 15 minutes or until lightly browned and tender. Cut the half avocado into slices.
2. Finally, in a large bowl layer the arugula, sprouts, avocado, and top with the tahini sauce. Enjoy the yummy taste.

Smoothie Recipes

Recipe 24: Pomegranate Smoothie

- Preparation Time: 10 minutes
- Total Servings: 2

Ingredients

- Pomegranate juice 1½ cups
- Water 1 cup
- Mixed berries 2 cups
- Thyme 2 tbsp.
- Lingonberries 1 oz.
- Ground flax seeds 1 tbsp.

Preparation Method

1. In a blender, place all ingredients and blend on medium speed until smooth.
2. Pour into a serving glass and enjoy.

Recipe 25: Aprines Smoothie

- Preparation Time: 10 minutes
- Servings per Recipe: 1

Ingredients

- Gingerroot 1 oz.
- Cinnamon 1 tbsp.
- Water 1 cup
- Nectarines 3½ oz.
- Apricot 2 oz.

Preparation Method

1. In a blender, place all the ingredients and blend on medium speed until smooth.
2. Pour into a serving glass and enjoy.

Recipe 26: Avocado Smoothie

- Preparation Time: 10 minutes
- Total Servings: 1

Ingredients

- Avocado 3 oz.
- Cranberry 3 oz.
- Lemon juice 1/3 cup
- Cinnamon 1 tsp.
- Water 1 cup

Preparation Method

1. In a blender, place all ingredients and blend on medium speed until smooth.
2. Pour into aserving glass and enjoy the taste.

Recipe 27: Vegetable Smoothie

- Preparation Time: 10 minutes
- Total Servings: 2

Ingredients

- Water 1 cup
- Half of an orange, peeled and seeds removed
- Baby carrots ¼ cup
- Cauliflower florets ¼ cup
- Broccoli florets ¼ cup
- Celery 1 stalk
- Lemon juice 1 tbsp.
- Dates, seed remove 1
- Chia seeds 1 tbsp.

Preparation Method

1. In a blender, place all ingredients and blend on medium speed until smooth.
2. Pour into 2 serving glasses and enjoy the taste.

Recipe 28: Super Green Smoothie

- Preparation Time: 10 minutes
- Total Servings: 2

Ingredients

- Kale 1½ cups
- Carrots 3 oz.
- Chopped celery 3 oz.
- Orange juice 1 cup
- Parsley 2 oz.
- Fresh Mint 2 oz.

Preparation Method

1. In a blender, place all ingredients and blend on medium speed until smooth.
2. Pour into serving glasses and enjoy.

Power-Pack Instant Energy Recipes

Recipe 29: Chicken Soup

- Preparation Time: 3 hours 10 minutes
- Total servings: 5

Ingredients

- Boneless chicken 1.2 lb.
- Onion Powder 1 tsp.
- Garlic Powder 1 tsp.
- Celery Seed ½ tsp.
- Ghee 2 oz.
- Acorn squash 1 oz.
- Chili sauce 2 oz.
- Chicken broth 3 cups
- Salt and Pepper to taste

Preparation Method

1. Cut the chicken into chunks and drop them into a crockpot. Add all the rest of the ingredients to the crockpot.
2. Set crockpot on high for 3 hours and cook completely. Once everything is cooked, remove the chicken from the crockpot and shred it using a fork
3. Add cream and cheese to the crockpot. Using an immersion blender, emulsify all of the liquids together. This will keep the soup from separating while you are eating
4. Place the chicken back into the crockpot and add cooked squash, stir together. Taste and season with extra salt, pepper, and chili sauce if needed. Serve and enjoy.

Recipe 30: Roasted Pears with Walnuts

- Preparation Time: 50 minutes
- Total servings: 4

Ingredients

- Pears 5
- Cinnamon powder 1 tsp.
- Cumin seeds 1 tsp.
- Walnut halves 2½ oz.
- Pine nuts 1 oz.

Optional

- Gingerroot 1 oz.

Preparation Method

1. Preheat the oven to 350°F. Peel the pears and cut them in half. Remove the core. Boil the pears in water for 2 minutes, Place the boiled pears in an oven-proof dish, sprinkle with cinnamon and bake for 20 min. or until they begin to brown. Remove from the oven and let them cool.
2. Toast the walnuts and pine nuts in the oven for 5 minutes. Save a few roasted pine nuts for garnish.
3. When the pears are cool,place them in a blender. blend pears, gingerroot, and roasted nuts until quite smooth and divide the pear mixture into 4 parts. Place on 4 serving dishes.
4. Finally, garnish each serving with chopped, roasted pine nuts and cumin seeds and serve immediately.

Recipe 31: Scrambled Spinach Tofu

- Preparation Time: 25 minutes
- Total servings: 2

Ingredients

- Tofu 14 oz.
- Ground turmeric ½ tsp.
- Salt to taste
- Freshly ground pepper to taste
- Cayenne pepper ½ tsp.
- Vegetable oil 2 tbsp.
- Sliced scallions 3
- Chopped spinach 5½ oz.
- Fresh lemon juice 2 tsp.
- Grape tomatoes 3½ oz.
- Basil, fresh, chopped 1 tbsp.

Preparation Method

1. In a medium bowl, mix tofu, black pepper, salt, and cayenne and set aside.
2. Place a pan over medium heat. Add oil and scallions, and cook until the scallions are soft. Add the tofu mixture and stir frequently until the tofu is brown — approximately 5 minutes.
3. Add the spinach, lemon juice, tomatoes and salt, and cook for 1 minute longer. Turn off the heat and garnish with the chopped basil. Serve and enjoy.

Recipe 32: Lentil Green salad

- Preparation Time: 30 minutes
- Total servings: 4

Ingredients

- Lentils 7-10 oz.
- Spring onions 1 bunch
- Cherry tomatoes 10 oz.
- Fresh flat-leaf parsley 1 bunch
- Fresh mint 1 bunch
- Vegetable oil 2 tbsp.
- Lemon juice 2 tbsp.
- Lemon zest 1 tsp.

Preparation Method

1. Rinse the lentils and boil them in salted water until tender. Drain and allow to cool.
2. Meanwhile, trim and finely chop the spring onions, halve the tomatoes, and chop the herb leaves.
3. Finally, mix the cool lentils with spring onions, tomatoes, herbs, vegetable oil, lemon juice, and zest. Season with salt and black pepper. Serve and enjoy this mouth-watering fresh herb salad.

Recipe 33: Three-Bean Chili

- Preparation Time: 30 minutes
- Total servings: 4

Ingredients

- Vegetable oil 1 tbsp.
- Onions ¼ cup (diced)
- Carrots ¼ cup (diced)
- Tomatoes 14 oz. (diced)
- Salt and black pepper to taste
- Chickpeas 15 oz.
- White beans 15 oz.
- Kidney beans 15 oz.
- Garlic powder 2 tsp.
- Nuts, chopped, 3 tbsp. (your choice)
- Fresh parsley 1 cup
- Water 2 cups
- Vegetable oil 2 tsp.
- Yogurt 1 tbsp.
- Optional: crisp bread

Preparation Method

1. Heat 1 tbsp. of the vegetable oil in a large pot over medium heat and add the onions and carrots. Cook, stirring, until tender; about 5 minutes.
2. Then add tomatoes, water, salt and pepper, and bring to a boil. After 5 minutes, add the chickpeas, white beans, and kidney beans and cook until heated; about 5 minutes.
3. In a small bowl, mix garlic, chopped nuts, parsley, 2 tsp. vegetable oil and salt. Divide the chili into 4 individual bowls and top with the yogurt. Serve with bread to enjoy extra taste.

Chapter 8: 21-Day Meal Plan

DAY	BREAKFAST	LUNCH	DINNER
Day 1	Avocado Omelet + Aprines Smoothie	Salmon with Mint Paste	Chicken Pumpkin Zoodles
Day 2	Almond Bars + Harvested Avocado Bowl	Baked Eggs with Kale	Dandelion Soup + Super Green Smoothie
Day 3	Avocado Omelet	Chicken Bone Soup	Summer Vegetable Stew
Day 4	Lemon Bread + Vegetable Smoothie	Green Herb Salad	Salmon Wraps
Day 5	Creamy Oatmeal	Mush-room Meal Plate	Dandelion Soup + Pome-granate Smoothie

Day 6	Pumpkin Bread + Broccoli Biscuits	Lentil Green salad	Chicken Soup
Day 7	Avocado Omelet	Chicken Bone Soup	Summer Vegetable Stew
Day 8	Creamy Oatmeal	Three-Bean Chili	Scrambled Spinach Tofu
Day 9	Lemon Bread + Vegetable Smoothie	Mush-room Meal Plate	Chicken Pumpkin Zoodles
Day 10	Creamy Oatmeal	Creamy Vegetable Soup	Roasted Pears with Walnuts
Day 11	Avocado Omelet	Veggie Salad	Chicken Pumpkin Zoodles
Day 12	Creamy Oatmeal	Roasted Pears with Walnuts	Three-Bean Chili
Day 13	Lemon Bread + Wild Mushroom Bowl	Chicken Bone Soup	Dandelion Soup

Day 14	Creamy Oatmeal	Macadamia Green Salad	Salmon Wraps
Day 15	Avocado Omelet	Creamy Vegetable Soup	Chicken Pumpkin Zoodles
Day 16	Creamy Oatmeal	Tuna Salad	Scrambled Spinach Tofu
Day 17	Pumpkin Bread	Chicken Bone Soup	Summer Vegetable Stew
Day 18	Avocado Omelet	Green Herb Salad	Dandelion Soup + Super Green Smoothie
Day 19	Creamy Oatmeal	Avocado Salad + Vegetable Smoothie	Summer Vegetable Stew
Day 20	Avocado Omelet	Creamy Vegetable Soup	Salmon Wraps
Day 21	Lemon Bread + Avocado Smoothie	Baked Eggs with Kale	Chicken Pumpkin Zoodles

Conclusion

The information provided in this book will help to educate you about the right path toward your goal to control and prevent diabetes, as well as to maintain good health throughout the rest of your life. Before you begin each day, remind yourself of the wonderful health benefits you can achieve while following our guide and remind yourself that improving your health and the environment is possible.